Science Experiments

SOUND AND HEARING

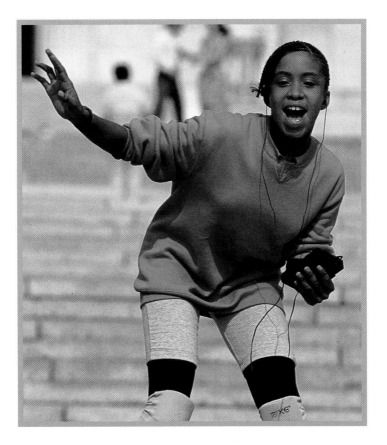

by
John Farndon

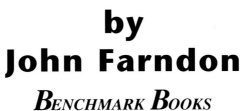

BENCHMARK BOOKS

MARSHALL CAVENDISH
NEW YORK

Marshall Cavendish Corporation
99 White Plains Road
Tarrytown, New York 10591
© Marshall Cavendish Corporation, 2001

Created by Brown Partworks Ltd

Library of Congress Cataloging-in-Publication Data
Farndon, John

    Sound and Hearing / by John Farndon
    p. cm. — (Science experiments)
    Includes index.
    Summary: A collection of experiments that explore the nature of
sound and how we hear it.
    ISBN 0-7614-1091-0 (lib. bdg.)
    1. Sound—Experiments—Juvenile literature. 2. Hearing—
Experiments—Juvenile literature. [1. Sound—Experiments. 2. Hearing—
Experiments. 3. Senses and sensation—Experiments. 4. Experiments.]
I. Title.

QC225.5 F37 2001   99-089262
534'.078—dc21

Printed in Hong Kong

PHOTOGRAPHIC CREDITS

t – top; b – bottom; c – center; l – left; r – right

Corbis: p4, Patrick Bennett (b); p16, James L.Amos (b); p17, Aron
Frankental (t); p20, 21 Joe McDonald (b); p22, 23 Randy Jolly (b);
p29, Perry Conway (br)
Duncan Brown: p26, 27(b)
The Image Bank: p8, 9 Cousteau Soc. (b); p24, Color Day (bl)
Image Select: p5,(br)
Pictor: title page; p12,(br)
SPL: p21, Saturn Stills (tr)

Step-by-step photography throughout: Martin Norris

Front cover: Martin Norris

Contents

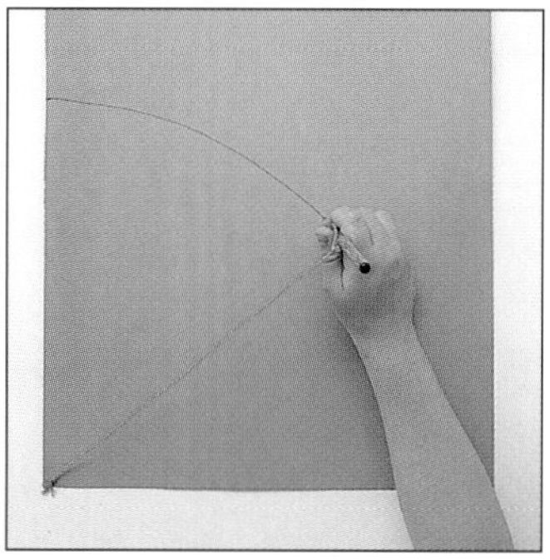

WHAT IS SOUND? — **4**

How to "See" Sounds — **6**

HOW SOUND MOVES — **8**

Making a String Telephone — **10**

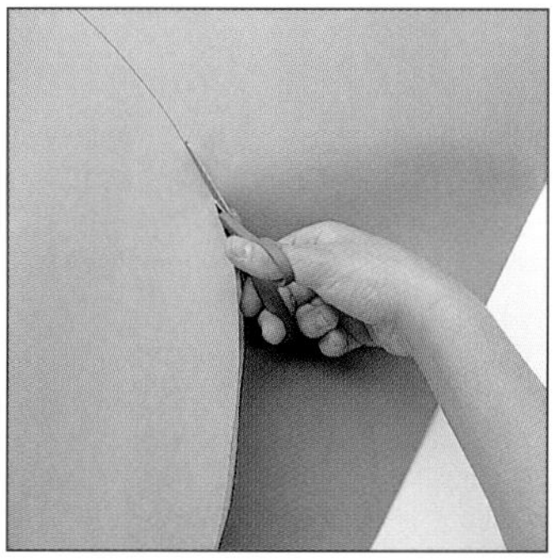

HOW WE HEAR SOUND — **12**

How to Make a Megaphone — **14**

PITCH: HIGH AND LOW — **16**

How to Make a Bottle Organ — **18**

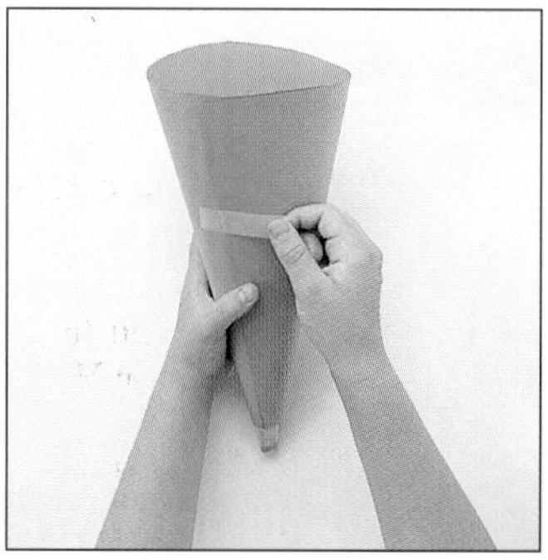

BEYOND HEARING — **20**

THE SPEED OF SOUND — **22**

Making Sound Change Pitch — **24**

BOUNCING SOUND — **26**

Games with Stereo Sound — **28**

Experiments in Science — **30**

Glossary — **31**

Index — **32**

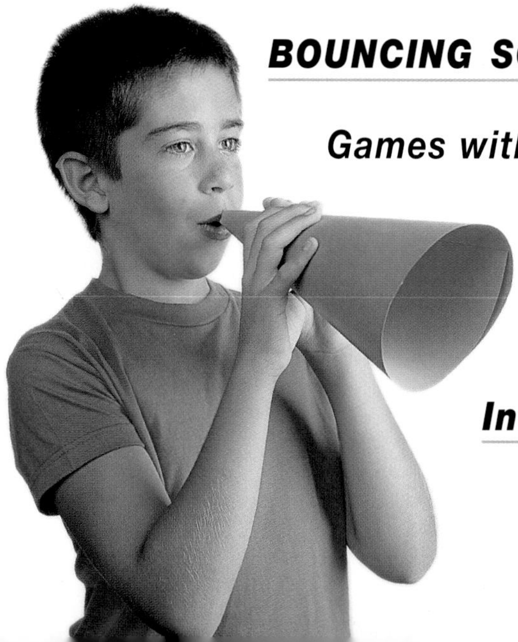

WHAT IS SOUND?

The roar of an aircraft taking off is one of the loudest sounds we hear.

The world is full of sound. Every time something moves, it makes a sound. Some sounds are very noisy, like an airplane taking off. Some—such as a fly's footsteps—are so soft that they can only be detected by the most sensitive instruments.

What all sounds, loud or quiet, have in common is that they are really air moving. When a dog barks, a violin is played, or the wind whispers in

Did you know?

Space is a vacuum beyond Earth's atmosphere. Sound cannot travel in a vacuum, so deep space is completely silent.

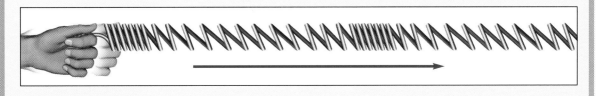

MAKING WAVES

You can see how sound waves move if you get a long soft spring. Place the spring, slightly stretched, on a very smooth, shiny surface, then give a sharp push at one end (above). You will see the coils cluster together, and the cluster appears to move down the spring with a corresponding stretching of coils behind. In the same way, when a sound is made, it is like a sharp shove on the air, and the air molecules near the sound are squashed together in clusters. They in turn push against the molecules next to them—and then are pulled back by the molecules behind them. Of course, each sound is not just one sharp shove on the air—but a whole series, one after another.

the grass, each makes the air vibrate, and these vibrations travel through the air and reach your ears. The vibrations are called sound waves. They are not like waves in the sea, which ripple across the water in lines. Sound waves move by alternately squeezing and stretching the air.

When a sound is made, molecules (all the tiny pieces of air) are squeezed together. As these molecules are pushed together, they squeeze on the molecules next to them and are pulled back into place by the molecules behind them. When the sound waves reach our ears, the ears pick up the vibrations, and the information is carried to our brains.

In the real world

SILENCE OF SPACE

If there are no molecules to move, sound cannot move either, so where there is no air, there can be no sound. Irish scientist Robert Boyle (1627–1691) proved this using a version of the air pump that had been devised by Otto von Guericke (1602–1686). Boyle pumped air out of a glass globe containing a loudly ticking watch. As he pumped out the air, creating a vacuum, the ticking became quieter. Eventually, he could see the watch's hands turning—but could hear no sound. When he let air back in the globe he could hear the ticking again.

Von Guericke used his air pump to create a vacuum—proving we need air to breathe.

HOW TO "SEE" SOUNDS

You will need

- ✔ A large round cake tin with a lid
- ✔ A large, strong elastic band
- ✔ A teaspoonful of colored sprinkles or granulated sugar
- ✔ A wooden spoon
- ✔ A plastic sheet

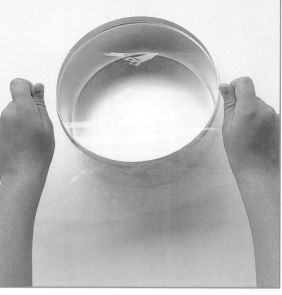

1 Take the lid off the tin and make a drum by stretching the plastic over the top, holding it in place with the elastic band.

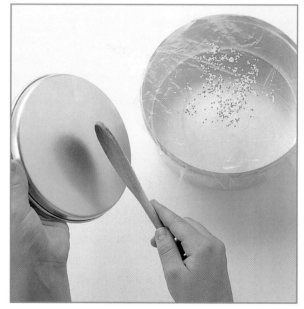

4 Hold the lid close to the tin and beat it with the wooden spoon. The sprinkles will dance up and down on the plastic.

Take it further

Sometimes you can see the movement that makes a sound. Pluck an elastic band, and you can see it twanging back and forth. Whistle and you see nothing. See if you can work out what it is that is vibrating to create different sounds. The sound of your voice is created by the vibration of the vocal cords in your throat as your breath passes over them. The sound of a guitar is made by the movement of the string. The sound of a bicycle bell is made by a little hammer in the bell hitting the metal dome.

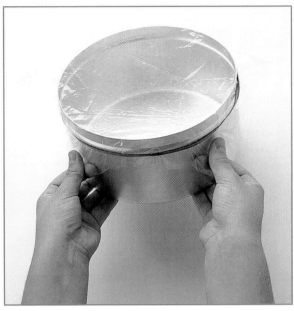

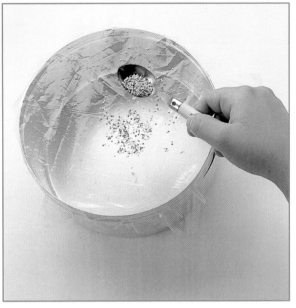

2 With the elastic band in place around the lip of the tin, pull the edges of the sheet out so that it is flat and tight.

3 Scatter a teaspoon or so of sprinkles carefully over the sheet, and spread the granules out evenly.

What is happening?

When you beat the tin lid, the shock makes the metal vibrate for a while afterward. As it vibrates, it sends out vibrations—sound waves—through the air. When the vibrations hit the plastic sheet, they set the sheet vibrating too, making the sprinkles dance. When the same vibrations reach your ear, you hear the sound of the wooden spoon hitting the tin lid.

HOW SOUND MOVES

Dolphins and other marine mammals use sound to communicate with each other through the water.

Most of the sounds we hear reach our ears through the air. But sound travels through other things as well—both solids and liquids. Only in a complete vacuum is there always complete silence, because sound cannot travel if there are no molecules to move. Sound travels especially well through liquids, because the molecules are packed close together. It is because of this that whales can communicate over huge distances in the sea. Whales use a mixture of low, booming sounds and high-pitched squeals to communicate with each other and find their way through the vast expanses of the oceans. Finback whales make a long, drawn-out sound,

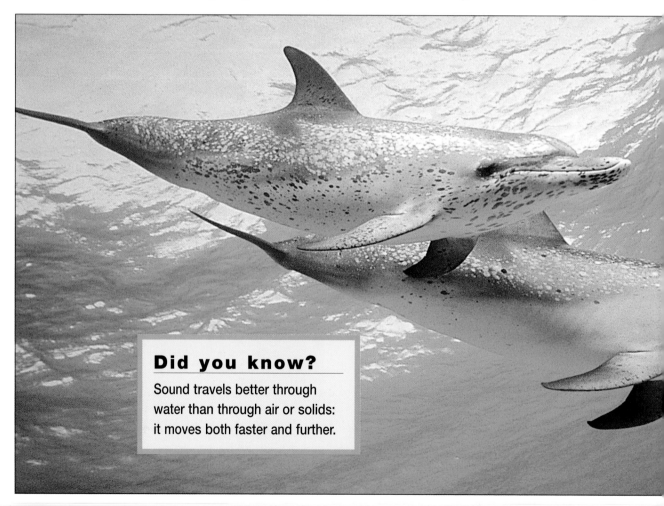

Did you know?

Sound travels better through water than through air or solids: it moves both faster and further.

which probably helps them keep in touch with each other even when they are over 500 miles (850 km) apart.

Sound travels through solids, but because the molecules in a solid are locked together, sound cannot move through a solid by stretching and squeezing the molecules as it does in the air. Sound travels best through solids that are so rigid—and thin—that the whole object moves back and forth. Metals ring and transmit high sounds clearly. Sand soaks up sound.

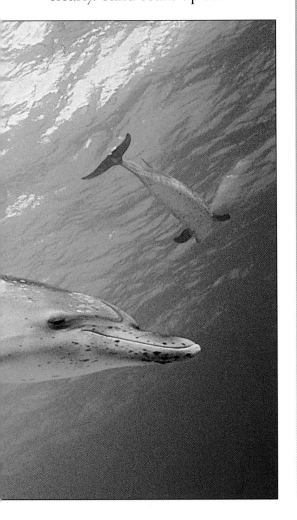

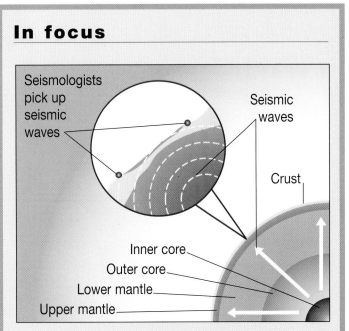

Seismologists pick up seismic waves

Seismic waves

Crust

Inner core
Outer core
Lower mantle
Upper mantle

LISTENING TO EARTH

We cannot see inside Earth—but we can hear. Whenever there is a big earthquake or a very loud underground explosion, the vibrations travel through Earth. In fact, many earthquake vibrations (scientists call them seismic waves) travel all the way through Earth and can be detected by sensitive instruments on the other side of the world.

Just as you can hear the difference between metal and wood if you tap it with a spoon, so scientists can "hear" what Earth's interior is made of by sending out their own seismic waves (above). Seismic waves are refracted (bent) as they pass through different materials and travel at different speeds. So scientists can work out what material the waves have passed through by timing their arrival. They have learned that Earth has only a thin rigid shell called the crust, then a very thick "mantle" of rock—over 1,600 miles (3,000 km) thick—so hot it is soft and almost molten. The very center of Earth is a core of metal.

Scientists have learned that the outer surface of the core is not smooth like a ball, but has continents, mountains, and valleys just like Earth's outer surface.

MAKING A STRING TELEPHONE

You will need

✔ A length of string about 20 ft (6 m) long

✔ Two identical empty tin cans with no sharp edges

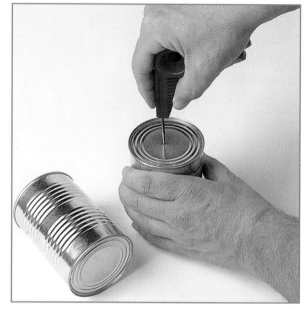

1 Get an adult to drill or punch a small hole in the bottom of each can, just big enough to thread the string through.

Take it further

Compare how well sound travels through the air and a solid. Try tapping on a table with your fingernail. Remember how loud the sound was as closely as you can. Now put your ear to the table so that you remain exactly the same distance away from your finger. Try tapping again. Is the sound louder or softer?

Try the same test on different materials: a carpeted floor, a tiled floor, a quilt, a mixing bowl, a mixing bowl full of water, a rubber tire, and a metal tray.

Now get a friend to tap on the far side of a wall when you have your ear to it. You will find out how well solids can transmit sound.

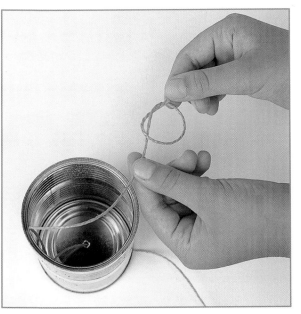

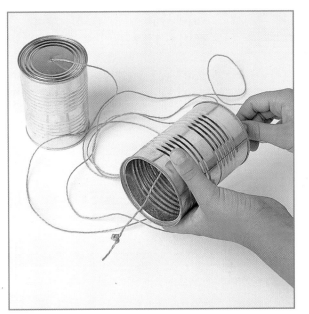

2 Thread one end of the string through the hole in one can, and tie a knot so that the string cannot slip back.

3 Thread the other end of the string through the bottom of the other can, then tie a knot as in the previous step.

What is happening?

Each different material transmits sounds in a different way. In this experiment the string is carrying the sound vibrations. You can see how effective this is by getting another person to stand the same distance away without the can—and see if he or she can hear your conversation.

You take one can and get a friend to take the other. Walk apart until the string is stretched taut. One of you try talking softly into the can. Take turns to speak and listen.

HOW WE HEAR SOUND

In stereo headphones, the earpieces create vibrations electrically.

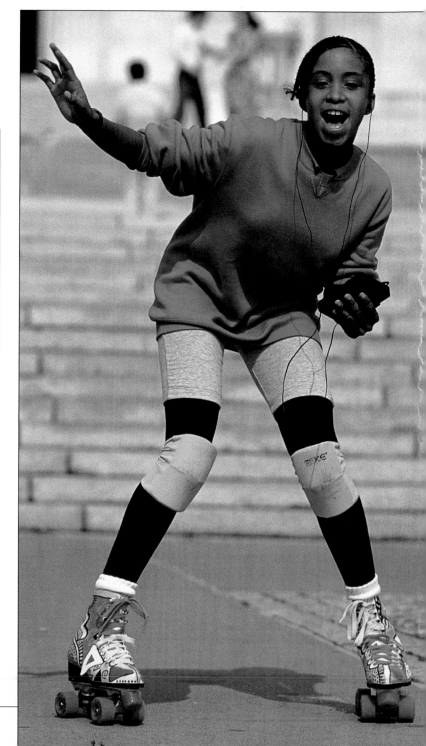

Did you know?

DEAFNESS

Usually only people born deaf are totally deaf. Most people who lose their hearing later in life—through disease, damage, or old age—can hear at least some sounds.

Hearing can go wrong in two ways. "Conductive" deafness occurs when the sound is not conducted (carried) properly from the outer ear to the inner ear. The problem may simply be a blockage of earwax, or the ear may be damaged by disease.

"Sensorineural" deafness is when the sound is not sent clearly from the inner ear to the brain—either because of damage to the inner ear or to the nerves carrying messages to the brain. The damage can be caused by very loud sounds.

Your ears are incredibly sensitive devices for picking up the tiny vibrations in the air that make up sounds.

Ears look simple, but the flap of skin on the outside of your head is just the entrance to the elaborate parts inside. The earflap simply funnels the vibrating air in toward the sensitive pressure detectors inside your head.

The ear actually has three sections: the outer, middle, and inner ear. The outer ear is the flap and the ear canal (the tunnel into your head). Inside your head, in the middle ear, the sound hits a taut membrane (a wall of skin) called the eardrum, shaking it rapidly. As the eardrum shakes, it rattles three tiny bones, or ossicles.

Even further inside, in the inner ear, is a curly tube called the cochlea, which is full of fluid. As the ossicles vibrate, they knock against this tube making waves in the fluid. The waves wash back and forth, and as they do, they push another membrane, called the organ of Corti, up and down so that it waggles some tiny, tiny hairs— almost like a hand playing the keys of a piano. As they waggle, the hairs send signals along the nerves to the brain.

In focus

INSIDE THE EAR

The air movements that make up each sound are so tiny that they must be made much bigger if the inner ear is to pick them up. So in the ear there are three small bones (ossicles) to make the movement stronger. The bones are all known by Latin names, which have English equivalents: the malleus or hammer, the incus or anvil, and the stapes or stirrup. When a sound vibrates the eardrum, the drum rattles the hammer against the anvil and the anvil shakes the stirrup. The hammer is the biggest of the bones, so it moves a long way with each vibration. The stirrup is the smallest and vibrates only a little way, but each vibration is much stronger than that of the hammer.

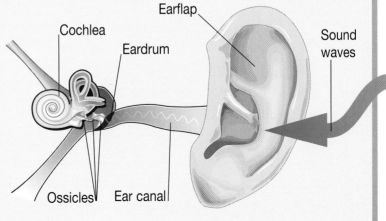

Earflap

Cochlea

Eardrum

Sound waves

Ossicles

Ear canal

HOW TO MAKE A MEGAPHONE

You will need

- ✔ A large sheet of thin card
- ✔ A piece of string, a pen, and a thumb tack
- ✔ Adhesive tape
- ✔ Scissors

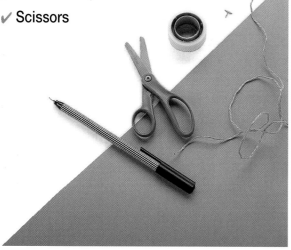

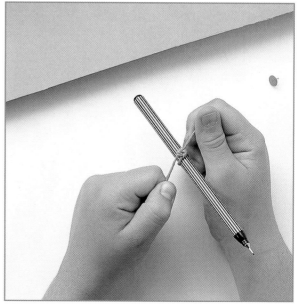

1 Tie the string to the thumb tack and the pen so that the length of the string is the same as the width of the card.

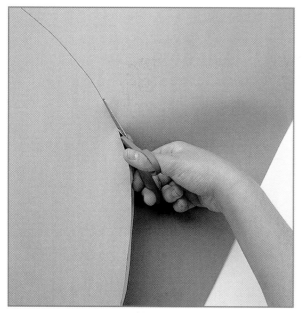

3 Draw a large curve on the card. Mark a small semicircle at the corner where the thumb tack was. Cut out the shape.

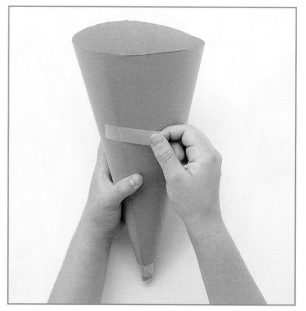

4 Roll the card so the edges overlap to form a cone. Use the adhesive tape to fix the free edge in place.

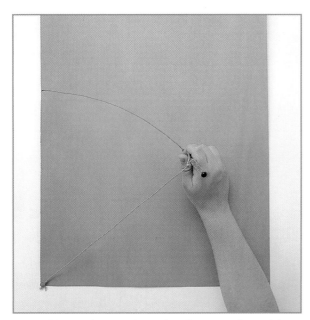

What is happening?

The shape of the megaphone makes the sound waves bounce, and the vibrations are made bigger and stronger. This makes the eardrum vibrate more, shaking the bones in the ear harder so that the sound seems louder. An electric megaphone makes the vibrations larger electrically.

2 Place the card on the floor and position the thumb tack at the corner of the card (pin it through into the carpet).

Hold the cone up to your lips and talk at a normal level. Ask a friend to test how much louder your voice sounds when you use the cone.

PITCH: HIGH AND LOW

Did you know?

The lowest sounds most people can make are about 80 Hz, but some singers have got down to 20.6 Hz. The highest sounds most people can make are 1,100 Hz, but some singers have got up to 4,350 Hz.

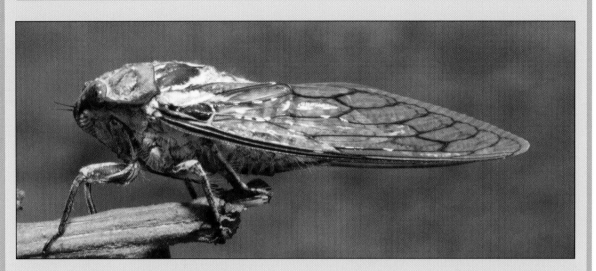

HIGH AND LOW SOUNDS

Sound frequency is usually measured in hertz (Hz), or cycles a second. Human ears can hear sounds from as low as 20 Hz up to as high as 20,000 Hz. The greater the frequency, the higher the pitch of a sound. Cicadas (above) make a chirping sound at about 120 Hz, which can be heard 1,800 ft (500 m) away.
- On average, men's voices are around 100 Hz.
- Women's voices are around 200 Hz.
- Children's voices are around 300 Hz.

Different instruments make noises at a different range of pitches: a bugle is quite high-pitched, while a tuba has a low pitch.

When you hear a bass drum booming or a rumble of thunder, you are hearing what is called a low-pitched sound. When you hear the squeal of brakes or tires, or a parrot screeching, you are hearing a high-pitched sound.

What makes these sounds different is, basically, the frequency of the sound waves that make them. The waves travel at exactly the same speed no matter what the pitch of the sound. What is different is how often they come. If the waves follow each other very quickly they make what is called a high-frequency sound, which is high in pitch. If they follow slowly, they make a low-frequency sound, which is low in pitch.

Although high-frequency waves come much faster after each other than low-frequency waves, the high-frequency waves are much shorter in length. Imagine an adult and small child walking together. If they walk at the same speed, the child has to take more steps (high-frequency steps) to keep up. The adult's steps are low in frequency.

HOW TO MAKE A BOTTLE ORGAN

You will need

✔ At least four identical small bottles, preferably with quite wide necks

✔ A measuring cup

✔ Food coloring

✔ Water

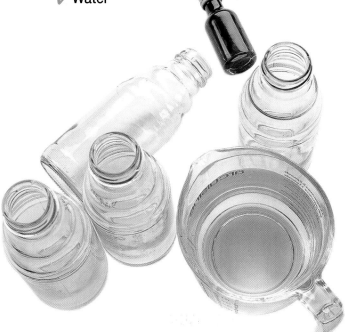

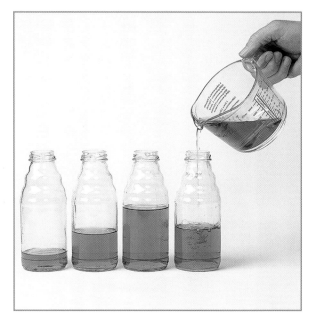

1 Use the measuring cup to pour increasing amounts of colored water into each of the glass bottles.

What is happening?

Like all sounds, music is simply air vibrating. Most pure musical notes are dominated by just a few different frequencies of vibration, at regular intervals. It is the regularity of the frequencies that makes a sound musical. The amount of space in the bottles affects the frequency of the vibrations, creating a series of different notes.

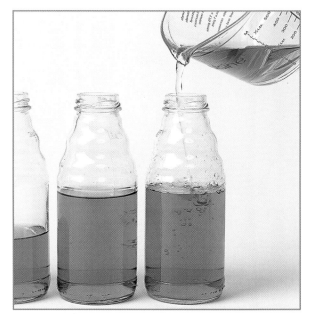

3 Try altering the amount of water in each bottle slightly, and see if you can create a proper musical scale of notes.

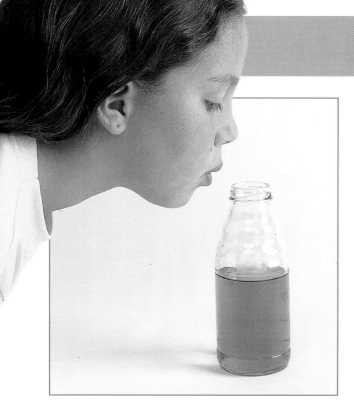

2 Blow across the top of a bottle to make a musical note. Blow across the others to see which makes the highest sound.

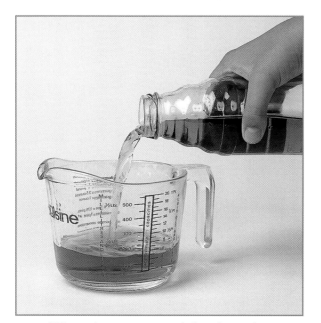

4 When the notes are right, does the amount of water in each bottle increase evenly? Measure it in the cup and see.

Take it further

MAKING MUSIC

STRING INSTRUMENTS like violins, cellos, and guitars make their sound with the vibration of a string. Different notes are made by pressing down on the string to make it shorter. Making it shorter makes it vibrate quicker and give a higher note.

BRASS INSTRUMENTS include trumpets and horns. The sound is made by the rapid vibration of the player's lips as he or she blows against the mouthpiece. The brass tube amplifies and refines the vibrations. Different notes are made either by blowing differently or with valves that change the inside length of the tube.

PERCUSSION INSTRUMENTS like drums and xylophones make a sound when they are shaken or hit. Most have a hollow space inside to make the sound resonate (bounce around).

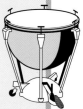

WIND INSTRUMENTS such as flutes and clarinets make their sound with a vibrating column of air inside a tube. To make the air vibrate, many have a "reed" in the mouthpiece—in the clarinet, for example, this is a thin slice of bamboo (reed), which vibrates when you blow.

BEYOND HEARING

Some sounds are just too high-pitched for the human ear to hear. These sounds are called ultrasounds. Yet although we cannot hear them, many animals can. While humans can only hear sounds as high as 20,000 Hz, dogs, for instance, can hear sounds as high as 50,000 Hz. Cats can hear sounds even higher.

Some animals rely on ultrasound for navigation and communication. Bats, for instance, find their way and keep in touch by emitting and listening for squeals at up to 120,000 Hz. Dolphins talk to

Bats navigate at night by using sound beyond hearing: they send out tiny squeaks, which bounce back to them, so that they can hear where they are going.

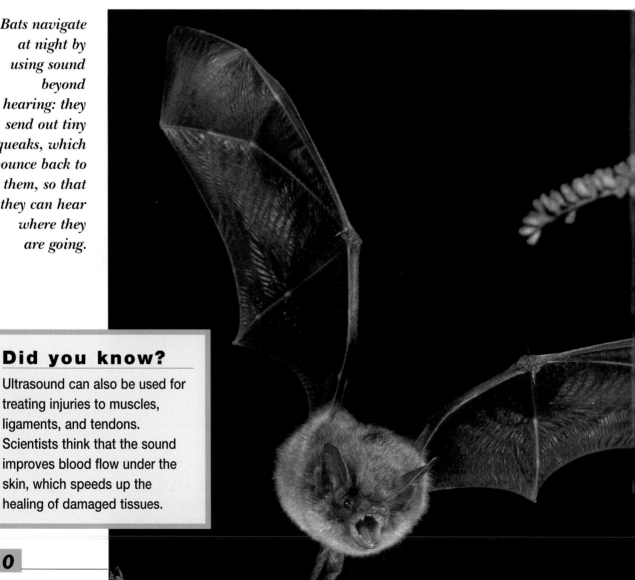

Did you know?

Ultrasound can also be used for treating injuries to muscles, ligaments, and tendons. Scientists think that the sound improves blood flow under the skin, which speeds up the healing of damaged tissues.

each other and locate each other using even higher clicks. These sounds are at least 120,000 Hz, and some scientists claim to have measured clicks at up to 280,000 Hz.

At the other end of the scale is infrasound—sound that is too low for the human ear to hear. Humans can hear as low as 20 Hz. Dogs can hear even lower sounds (down to 15 Hz), and whales communicate with very low rumbles.

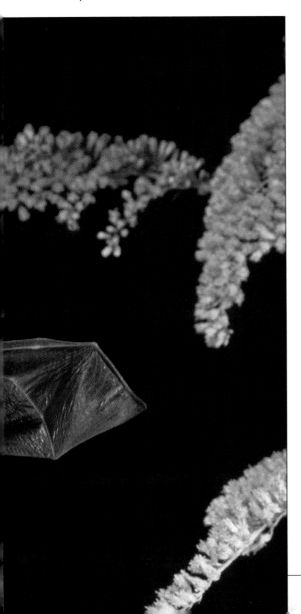

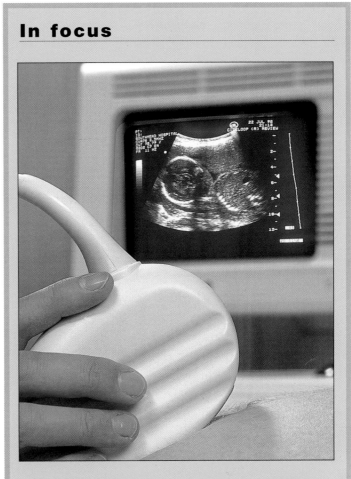

INSIDE THE WOMB

Ultrasound penetrates certain materials much better than normal frequency sound. In fact, it penetrates bodies so well that doctors can use it to look inside an expectant mother's body to check on how the baby is developing inside her womb.

Ultrasound scans use a device called a transducer (above) to send out sound at 1 to 15 million Hz—sounds so high they can be focused into a narrow beam. The sound beam is reflected back from different depths within the body, according to the different materials (bone and skin) that it meets. A detector picks up the pattern of reflections and converts the signals into pictures to display on a screen. The pictures are fuzzy, but clear enough to see the outline of the baby inside—and see it moving.

THE SPEED OF SOUND

When you're talking to someone, their voice seems to reach you instantly. But sounds actually take time to move through the air. Watch a piledriver pound down on a distant building site and you will hear the thud marginally after you see the hammer go down. In a thunderstorm, you may hear the rumble of thunder several seconds after you see the flash of lightning that caused it.

The speed at which sound travels actually varies a little depending on how warm or cold the air is. In air at 70°F (20°C), the speed of sound is 1,130 ft (343 m) per second. If it is very hot, 110°F (40°C), the speed of sound is slightly faster, at 1,161 ft (354 m) per second. At freezing point, it travels at 1,086 ft (331 m) per second.

This fighter jet can fly faster than the speed of sound: you would not hear it until it had flown over you.

In focus

Supersonic jets fly faster than the speed of sound. You cannot hear them coming—the jet passes by before the sound reaches you.

When pilots first tried to fly faster than sound, they found that as a jet approached the speed of sound, it is buffeted by shock waves. The reason is that the plane catches up with the sound waves radiating in front of it—and squeezes them up to form shock waves, which rock the plane. Eventually, the plane overtakes these shock waves, breaking the "sound barrier" and leaving a sonic boom behind.

Did you know?

The speed at which supersonic aircraft travel is often given in terms of Mach numbers, after the Austrian physicist Ernst Mach (1838–1916) who first described how supersonic shock waves are formed. A plane flying at the speed of sound is said to be flying at Mach 1. A plane flying at twice the speed of sound is flying at Mach 2.

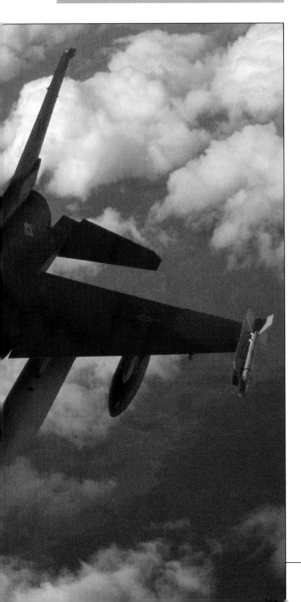

Now try this

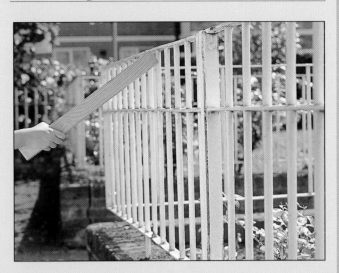

TESTING SOUND SPEED

Sound travels much faster in water, at a rate of 4,820 ft per second (1,483 m per second) at 70°F (20°C), and even faster in solids—traveling at 13,000 ft per second (4,000 m per second) in wood and almost 20,000 ft per second (6,000 m per second) in steel. You can hear this by getting a friend to tap a long, straight iron railing (above). Put your ear to the railing at the other end (below). You will hear two separate sounds: first the sound reaches your ear through the railing, then it arrives through the air.

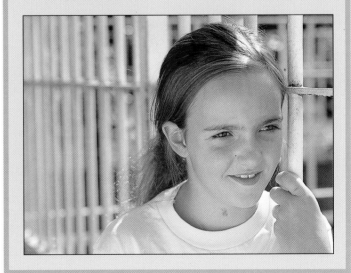

MAKING SOUND CHANGE PITCH

You will need

✔ A whistle
✔ A bicycle

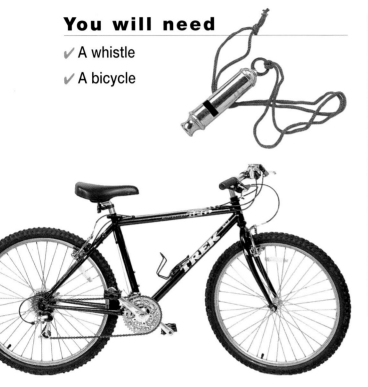

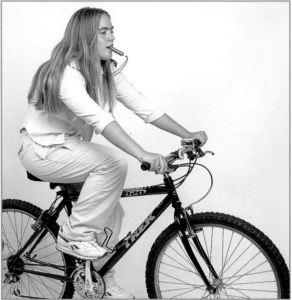

1 Get your friend to cycle past you very slowly blowing the whistle continuously. Listen carefully for any change of pitch in the whistle. You will probably hear none.

In the real world

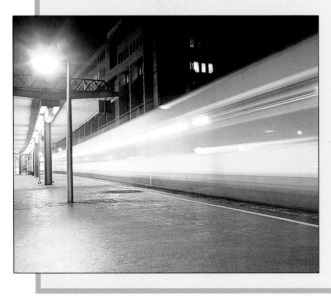

MOVING SOUND

Listen carefully to the sound of a train running through a station (left), a car speeding down the road, or a police siren screeching past, and you will hear something odd happen to the pitch of the sound. You might expect it to stay the same since it comes from the same source. In fact, as the train gets nearer the sound seems to get higher—and then lower again as the train passes by. This effect is known as the Doppler effect after the Austrian physicist Christian Doppler (1803–1853) who first noticed it about 150 years ago.

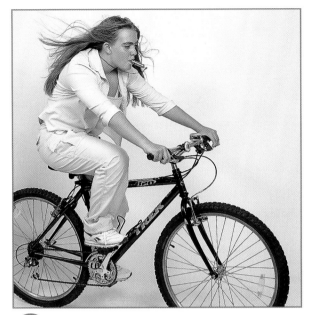

As the bicycle and the sound of the whistle approach, the waves are squeezed together, making them higher in frequency, and so they are a higher pitch. As it goes away from you, the waves stretch apart, so the sound is lower in pitch.

2 Now get your friend to whizz by you as quickly as possible, blowing the whistle steadily. Listen for the rising and falling of the pitch of the whistle.

In focus

The same Doppler effect happens with light traveling through space as with sound. Distant galaxies are moving away from us so fast that the waves of light they send out are stretched out, just like the sound waves behind a receding car.

When light waves are stretched out, they don't drop in pitch, they go redder. So this effect is called red shift.

Astronomers can tell just how fast a galaxy is moving away from the degree of red shift—that is, how much redder the light from the galaxy is than they would expect it to be.

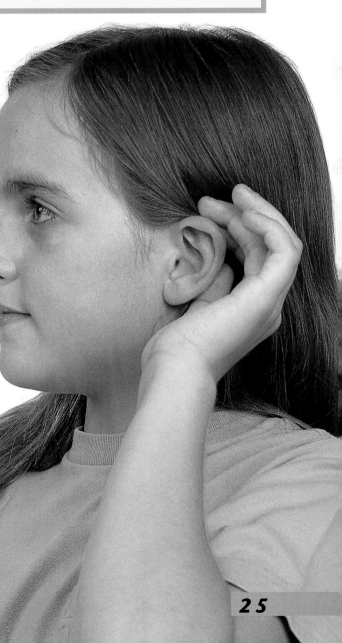

BOUNCING SOUND

Shout in a large, empty hall or a under a bridge and you can often hear the sound of your voice ringing out a moment or two afterward.

This is an echo—it is just your voice bouncing back off the walls. Sound bounces off every smooth hard wall, near or far. In a small room it bounces back so quickly that you cannot distinguish it from the original sound. But if the wall is some distance away, the sound takes a little time to get back to you, so it overlaps with, or repeats, the

Concert halls, such as Sydney Opera House, Australia, are carefully designed for the best acoustics.

original sound. You can only hear an echo if the sound comes back at least 0.1 second after the original sound. Since sound travels about 100 ft (30 m) in 0.1 second, you only hear echoes from surfaces at least 50 ft (15 m) away.

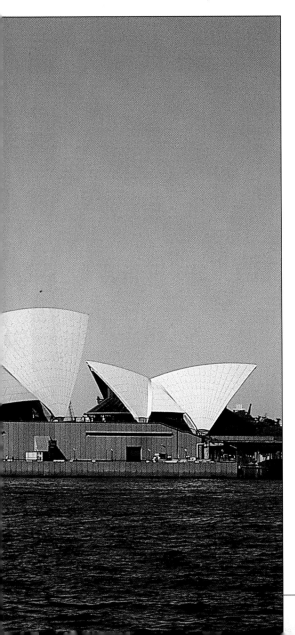

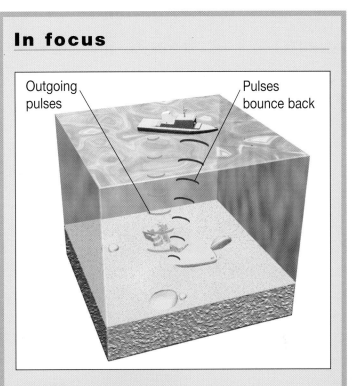

Outgoing pulses

Pulses bounce back

SOUND MAPPING

Because sound travels so well in water, ships can use echoes to pinpoint shoals of fish, detect submarines, and chart the depths of the ocean. Sonar (*s*ound *n*avigation *a*nd *r*anging) equipment sends out pulses of high-frequency pings, generated electronically. The time it takes for the sound pulse to bounce back from unseen objects up to 6 miles (10 km) away indicates how far away the objects are.

Oceanographers (scientists who study the oceans) are using sonar, often from robot submarines, to build up a detailed map of the ocean floor for the first time. Their discoveries have revealed that the ocean bed is a landscape as fascinating and varied as the continents. For example, they showed that along the middle of the Atlantic Ocean winds a mountain ridge 25,000 miles (40,000 km) long—the world's longest mountain range.

Sonar has other uses too: many fascinating shipwrecks such as Henry VIII's *Mary Rose* and the *Titanic* would not have been found without sonar.

GAMES WITH STEREO SOUND

You will need

✔ Objects for making various different noises such as a comb, a piece of paper, some potato chips, a small bell

✔ A blindfold

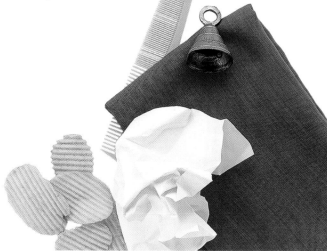

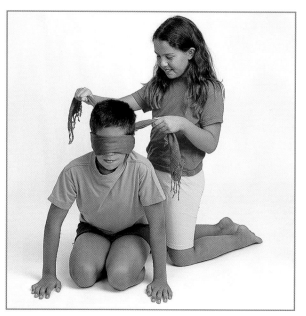

1 Go into a large, relatively empty room and sit in the middle. Ask a friend to help you tie a blindfold over your eyes.

Take it further

SLEEPING PIRATE

• One person sits blindfolded, beside a "treasure" on the floor. All the others sit around in silence, in a circle about 20 ft (6 m) across.

• A person is picked to make the first raid. Her task is to sneak up slowly and quietly, a step at a time and steal the treasure.

• The "sleeping pirate" in the middle has to listen for the raider's footsteps, and point to the sound. If the pirate points to the raider, the raider has failed—another raider takes a turn.

• The game goes on until a raider reaches the treasure without being heard.

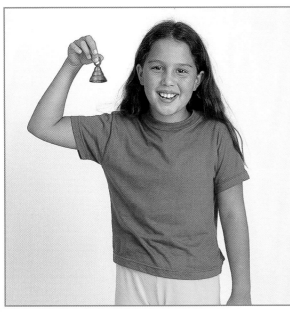

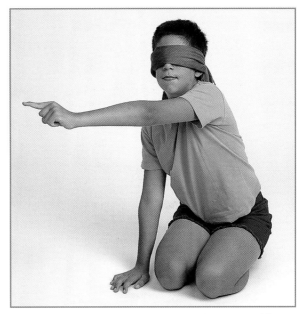

2 Ask your friend to use the different objects to make quiet sounds from different parts of the room.

3 Point to where you think the sound is coming from. Let your friend judge how accurate you are.

What is happening?

When you hear a sound you hear it in stereo: the sound waves bounce around the room and reach one ear a fraction of a second after they reach the other and are very slightly quieter—unless the sound is directly in front of you. The further to one side the source of the sound is, the bigger will be the delay between one ear and the other. Your brain interprets the slight delay, and the difference in the sound, to pinpoint just where the sound is coming from.

Most animals have two ears to help them pinpoint sounds, but some animals are better at it than others. Owls (right) are so good at it that they can use it to find a running mouse in the pitch dark of a forest at night.

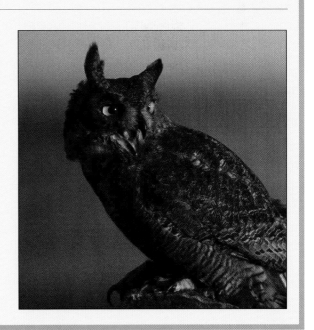

Experiments in Science

Science is about knowledge: it is concerned with knowing and trying to understand the world around us. The word comes from the Latin word, *scire*, to know.

In the early 17th century, the great English thinker Francis Bacon (1521–1626) suggested that the best way to learn about the world was not simply to think about it, but to go out and look for yourself—to make observations and try things out. Ever since then, scientists have tried to approach their work with both observation and experiment. Scientists insist that an idea or theory must be thoroughly tested before it is widely accepted.

All the experiments in this book have been tried before, and the theories behind them are widely accepted. But that is no reason why you should accept them. Once you have done all the experiments in this book, you will know the ideas are true not because we have told you so, but because you have seen for yourself.

All too often in science there is an external factor interfering with the result which the scientist just has not thought of. Sometimes this can make the experiment seem to work when it has not, as well as making it fail. One scientist conducted lots of demonstrations to show that a clever horse called Hans could count things and tap out the answer with his hoof. The horse was indeed clever, but later it was found that rather than counting, he was getting clues from tiny unconscious movements of the scientist's eyebrows.

This is why it is very important when conducting experiments to be as rigorous as you possibly can. The more casual you are, the more "eyebrow factors" you will let in. There will always be some things that you cannot control. But the more precise you are, the less these are likely to affect the outcome.

What went wrong?

However careful you are, your experiments may not work. If so, you should try to find out where you went wrong. Then repeat the experiment until you are absolutely sure you are doing everything right. Scientists learn as much, if not more, from experiments that go wrong as those that succeed. In 1929, Alexander Fleming (1881–1955) discovered the first antibiotic drug, penicillin, when he noticed that a bacteria culture he was growing for an experiment had gone moldy—and that the mold seemed to kill the bacteria. A poor scientist would probably have thrown the moldy culture away. A good scientist is one who looks for alternative explanations for unexpected results.

Glossary

Absorption: The opposite of radiation—the soaking up of light, heat, sound, and other forms of energy.

Acoustics: The science of sound. In particular, acoustics looks at the way sound is transmitted in buildings, sound systems, and musical instruments.

Doppler effect: The change in the apparent length of a wave of sound or light as its source moves toward or away from you. You can hear it in the rise and fall in pitch in the sound of a car zooming past. Astronomers see it in the redder color or "red shift" of galaxies moving away from Earth.

Echo: A reflected sound or radio signal.

Frequency: The number of waves of sound per second, usually measured in waves or cycles per second, known as Hertz (Hz). The pitch of a musical note is its frequency.

Infrasound: Sound too low in pitch for humans to hear.

Mach scale: A scale for describing how fast an aircraft is traveling compared to the speed of sound, named for Austrian physicist Ernst Mach (1838–1916).

Pitch: The "highness" or "lowness" of one sound compared to another.

Refraction: The change in direction that waves undergo when they pass through the barrier between materials, in which the waves move at different speeds. For example, light is refracted when it travels through the barrier between air and water, which is why a pencil in a glass of water appears bent.

Reverberation: Sound that has undergone lots of echoes.

Seismologist: A scientist who studies earthquakes.

Sonic boom: The loud noise caused by the shock waves made by an aircraft traveling faster than the speed of sound.

Sound barrier: The barrier of shock waves that a plane must overtake in order to fly faster than the speed of sound.

Speed of sound: This is the speed at which sound travels. It is different depending on what material the sound is traveling through.

Supersonic: Anything that can travel faster than the speed of sound, including airplanes.

Ultrasound: Sound too high in pitch to be heard by human ears.

Vacuum: A space that contains nothing at all; no air, no water, no matter, just empty space.

Index

A, B, C

acoustics 26
Boyle, Robert 5
cicada 17
cochlea 13
conductive deafness 12
Corti, organ of 13
crust, of Earth 9

D, E, F, G

deafness 12
dolphins 20
Doppler, Christian 24
Doppler effect 24
ear 13
eardrum 13, 15
earwax 12
echo 26
frequency 17, 18, 25
Guericke, Otto von 5

H, I, J, K

hearing in bats 20
hearing in dogs 20
hearing in owls 29
high frequency 17
infrasound 21
injuries to muscles, ligaments, and
        tendons 20
inner ear 13

L, M, N, O

liquids, sound travels through 8, 23
low frequency 17
Mach 1, Mach 2 23
Mach, Ernst 23

mantle 9
megaphone 14, 15
middle ear 13
musical instruments 19
oceanographer 27
ossicles 13
outer ear 13

P, Q, R, S

pitch 17, 25
red shift 25
seismic waves 9
seismologist 9
sensorineural deafness 12
shock waves 22
solids, sound travels through 9, 10, 23
sonar 27
sonic boom 22
sound, speed of 22
sound waves 5, 13
space 4, 25
stereo 28, 29
Sydney Opera House 26

T, U, V

transducer 21
ultrasound 20, 21
vacuum 4, 8
vibration(s) 5, 7, 11, 13, 18, 19
vocal cords 6
vortex 18

W, X, Y, Z

waves, seismic 9
waves, shock 22
waves, sound 5, 13